BLOOD TYPE A

FOOD, BEVERAGE AND SUPPLEMENT LISTS

from

EAT RIGHT

F4R

YOUR TYPE

Dr. Peter J. D'Adamo
with Catherine Whitney

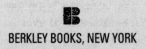

BERKLEY BOOKS, NEW YORK

BLOOD TYPE A: FOOD, BEVERAGE AND SUPPLEMENT LISTS

Every effort has been made to ensure that the information contained in this book is complete and accurate. However, neither the publisher nor the authors are engaged in rendering professional advice or services to the individual reader. The ideas, procedures, and suggestions contained in this book are not intended as a substitute for consulting with your physician. All matters regarding your health require medical supervision. Neither the authors nor the publisher shall be liable or responsible for any loss, injury, or damage allegedly arising from any information or suggestion in this book. The opinions expressed in this book represent the personal views of the authors and not of the publisher.

A Berkley Book / published by arrangement with
the authors

PRINTING HISTORY
Berkley edition / January 2002

All rights reserved.
Copyright © 2002 by Hoop-A-Joop, LLC
Book design by Tiffany Kukec
Cover design by Steven Ferlauto
This book, or parts thereof, may not be reproduced in any form without permission. For information address: The Berkley Publishing Group, a division of Penguin Putnam Inc., 375 Hudson Street, New York, New York 10014.

ISBN: 0-425-18311-4

BERKLEY®
Berkley Books are published by The Berkley Publishing Group, a division of Penguin Putnam Inc., 375 Hudson Street, New York, New York 10014.
BERKLEY and the "B" design
are trademarks belonging to Penguin Putnam Inc.

PRINTED IN THE UNITED STATES OF AMERICA

20 19 18 17

*To Blood Type As of the
Twenty-first Century, that you may fully realize
your remarkable heritage.*

Contents

Acknowledgments

There are many people to thank, as no scientific pursuit is solitary. Along the way, I have been driven, inspired, and supported by all of the people who placed their confidence in me. In particular, I give deep thanks to my wife, Martha, for her love and friendship; my daughters, Claudia and Emily, for the joy they bring me; and my parents, James D'Adamo Sr., N.D., and Christl, for teaching me to trust in my intuition.

I am also more grateful than I can express to:

Catherine Whitney, my writer, and her partner, Paul Krafin, who have transformed complex scientific ideas into accessible principles of everyday life;

My literary agent, Janis Vallely, whose commitment and wisdom are a continuing aid and inspiration;

Amy Hertz, my editor at Riverhead/Putnam, whose

vision and care have turned the blood type science into a meaningful mainstream program;

Jane Dystel, Catherine's literary agent, whose advice has been welcome;

Heidi Merritt, whose devotion and attention to detail have brought the manuscript closer to perfection;

My staff at 2009 Summer Street for their dedication and support, and the hardworking staff at 5 Brook Street;

All of the wonderful patients who in their quest for health and happiness chose to honor me with their trust.

What Type As Are Saying About the Diet

From Mary T., 52:

"I have been roller-coaster dieting for the past 20 years and have lost and regained hundreds of pounds. I was at 200 pounds when I started the diet in March. I am now at 165 and still losing. There were several reasons why I decided to do this diet, but the main one was that my normally slim, runner husband had begun to gain weight and had no energy. I had been trying to get him on a lower-fat diet for about a year, and this diet intrigued him. We are both Type A, so it was quite easy to do. Within four days of no dairy, my husband stopped snoring. I moved back into our bedroom from the guest room. I have gone from a size 18 to a size 12, and my husband is in size 34 pants for the first time since high school. He lost 25 pounds in about six weeks. Most significant is that his triglycerides went from 608 to 177 in two months. And we are not starving ourselves in the least."

From Ned K., 35:

"I suffered from chronic irritable bowel syndrome, but since embracing the plan for Type A, my life has changed dramatically. I cannot even believe the difference. I had been to GI doctors, had countless tests done, and was basically told there was nothing to be done about it. It was unacceptable to me, at age 34, to be facing the lifelong prospect of constantly irritated bowels. When I switched to the Type A Diet, I could not believe the difference. It was and is truly amazing. I have shared my findings with friends and family members, and have already been told by both my mother and brother that they, too, are experiencing a great degree of success with the plan. Thank you so much. You can't even imagine how much I appreciate your findings and research."

From Rena W., 37

"This diet has completely changed me inside and out! I started the diet after I was diagnosed with polycystic ovarian disease. I knew I had to get serious about my health and weight. I am pleased to say now that I have lost 25 pounds. I have seen a huge improvement in my health as well. I truly believe that this is the diet everyone should use! One day the world and doctors will realize this."

From Helen S., 33

"I have lost 15 pounds in two months, which is great in itself, but there is more. I have the most amazing sense of well being that I have ever had. This is especially spectacular when you realize

that I am a stay-at-home mom with kids screaming 24/7. A true test of my energy came at Disneyland. Even losing the weight that I had, I still outlasted the other four adults I was with."

From Bruce E., 54

"Lab tests indicate a dramatic decrease in my blood cholesterol and triglycerides since I started the Type A Diet. I've also lost more than 20 pounds, my digestion is working much better, my energy is more stable throughout the day, and my thinking is clearer. Everything got better on the plan. I practice acupuncture and herbal medicine and regularly recommend this to my patients."

From Stephanie S., 29

"I successfully followed the principles for Blood Type A for approximately four months and experienced tremendous health benefits. My mucus was gone (amazing), I lost 10 pounds in three months, and felt right with my body for the first time in years. However, when I went through a period of fatigue nine months after starting the diet, I decided that based on the recent hoopla, I should eat a high-protein diet. I gobbled meat, cheese, heavy creams, and high-fat nuts with some lettuce in between. After a week, I'd gained five pounds, felt sullied from all that meat, and confused. All of the high-protein plans claim that the pounds just fall off, but for me it was the opposite. Must be all those Type Os creating the rave. I'm back on Type A foods, and I toast my soy milk latte to Dr. D'Adamo."

A Message for Type As

Dear Type A Reader,

This special-format book, Eat Right 4 Type A, *focuses on the principles and strategies of the Blood Type Diet as they apply to you. If you are new to the diet, you'll find this book to be a simple, accessible beginner's guide that will get you started on the basics. If you are already following the diet and have read the comprehensive series (*Eat Right 4 Your Type, Cook Right 4 Your Type, *and* Live Right 4 Your Type*), you'll find this book useful as a quick and portable reference guide for your diet.*

Since the introduction of the Blood Type Diet five years ago, I have received tens of thousands of testimonials from people all over the world. Many of them are from Type As who have overcome chronic health problems, serious illnesses, or lifelong struggles with weight

merely by eating and living in accordance with the ge-
netic signals of their blood type. A growing body of re-
search supports the conclusion that our individual
differences do *matter when it comes to making strategic*
health and lifestyle decisions.

I sincerely hope that you will join other Type As who
have had success with this plan. I invite you to share in
experiencing the renewed sense of well-being and good
health that have become reliable hallmarks of the Type
A Diet.

Peter J. D'Adamo, N.D.

IMPORTANT NOTE

The contents of this book have been abridged to provide only the most basic information concerning the Blood Type Diet. To gain the full therapeutic benefit of the diet, it is important that you read Dr. D'Adamo's complete research and prescriptive advice as it appears in his three books, *Eat Right 4 Your Type, Cook Right 4 Your Type* and *Live Right 4 Your Type*. These books include extensive details that will help you fully understand the important role your blood type plays in determining diet, exercise, health, disease, longevity, physical vitality, and emotional stability.

The Blood Type–Diet Connection

The connection between blood type and diet is a new idea for most people, but they often find that it answers some of their most perplexing questions. We have long realized that there was a missing link in our comprehension of the process that leads either to the path of wellness or the path of disease. There had to be a reason why there were so many paradoxes in dietary studies and disease survival. Blood type analysis has given us a way to explain those paradoxes.

Blood types are as fundamental as creation itself. In the masterful logic of nature, the four blood types follow an unbroken trail from the earliest moment of human creation to the present day. They are the signatures of our ancient ancestors on the indestructible parchment of history. The gene for Blood Type A emerged at a point in history when humans were evolving from hunter-gatherers and settling into more permanent agrarian communities. The Type A gene enabled your ancestors to survive and thrive on a vegetarian-based diet. Amazingly, at the beginning of the twenty-first century, your immune and digestive systems still maintain a predisposition for foods that your Type A ancestors ate.

Your blood type is the key to your body's entire immune system, and as such is the essential defining factor in your health profile. Your blood type antigen serves as the guardian at the gate, creating antibodies to ward off dangerous interlopers. When an antibody encounters the antigen of a microbial invader, a reaction called "agglutination" (literally, gluing) occurs. The antibody attaches to the viral antigen and makes it very sticky. When cells, viruses, parasites, and bacteria are agglutinated, they stick together and clump up, which makes the job of their disposal all the easier.

But there is much more to the agglutination story. Scientists have learned that many foods agglutinate the cells of certain blood types but not others, meaning that a food that may be harmful to the cells of one blood type may be beneficial to the cells of another.

A chemical reaction occurs between your blood and the foods that you eat. This reaction is part of your genetic inheritance. We know this because of a factor called "lectins." Lectins, abundant and diverse proteins found in foods, have agglutinating properties that affect your blood. Lectins are a powerful way for organisms in nature to attach themselves to other organisms in nature. Often, the lectins used by viruses or bacteria can be blood type specific, making them a stickier pest for a person of that blood type. Furthermore, when you eat a food containing protein lectins that are incompatible with your blood type antigen, the lectins target an organ or bodily system (kidneys, liver, brain, stomach, etc.) and begin to agglutinate blood cells in that area. For example, the lectin in lima beans cross-reacts with the Type A antigen, targeting digestive enzymes and interfering with insulin production.

The Type A Diet is a way to restore the natural protective functions of your immune system, reset your metabolic clock, and clear your blood of dangerous agglutinating lectins. Depending on the severity of the condition, and the level of compliance with the plan, every person will realize some benefits from this diet.

THE TYPE A DIET BASICS

Type As flourish on vegetarian diets—the inheritance of your more settled and less warlike farmer ancestors. If you are an average American with Type A blood, you might find it a big adjustment to move away from the typical meat and potato fare to soy proteins, grains, and vegetables. Likewise, you may find it difficult to eliminate overly processed and refined foods, since our civilized diets are increasingly composed of convenient toxins in brightly wrapped packages. But it is particularly important for sensitive Type As to get your foods in as natural a state as possible: fresh, pure, and organic. If you follow the Type A Diet, you can supercharge your immune system and potentially short-circuit the development of life-threatening diseases. A positive aspect of your genetic ancestry is your ability to utilize the best nature has to offer. It will be your challenge to relearn what your blood already knows.

The Type A Diet works because you are able to follow a clear, logical, scientifically researched and certified dietary blueprint based on your cellular profile.

Your diet is organized into fourteen food groups:

Meats and Poultry	**Vegetables**
Seafood	**Fruits**
Eggs and Dairy	**Juices and Fluids**
Oils and Fats	**Spices**
Nuts and Seeds	**Condiments**
Beans and Legumes	**Herbs and Herbal Teas**
Grains, Breads and Pasta	**Miscellaneous Beverages**

Within each group, food is divided into three categories: HIGHLY BENEFICIAL, NEUTRAL, and AVOID. Think of the categories this way:

- **HIGHLY BENEFICIAL** is a food that acts like a **MEDICINE**.

- **AVOID** is a food that acts like a **POISON**.

- **NEUTRAL** is a food that acts like a **FOOD**.

The Type A Diet includes a wide variety of foods, so don't worry about limitations. When possible, show preference for the Highly Beneficial foods over the Neutral foods, but feel free to enjoy the Neutral foods that suit you; they won't harm you and they contain nutrients that are necessary for a balanced diet.

At the top of each food category, you will see a chart that looks something like this (note that the frequency is sometimes weekly, sometimes daily):

		Weekly, if your ancestry is . . .		
BLOOD TYPE A	PORTION	AFRICAN	CAUCASIAN	ASIAN
All seafood	4–6 oz.	1–4 x	3–5 x	4–6 x

The portion suggestions according to ancestry are not meant as firm rules. My purpose here is to present a way to fine-tune your diet even more, using what is known about the particulars of your ancestry. Although peoples of different races and cultures may share a blood type, they don't always have the same frequency of the gene. For example, a Type A person may be AA, meaning both parents passed on the A gene, or AO, meaning only one parent passed on the A gene. Overall, people of African ancestry tend to carry the O gene more frequently than people of Caucasian and Asian ancestry. There are also geographic and cultural variations, as well as typical differences in the size and weight of various peoples.

Use the refinements if you think they're helpful; ignore them if you find that they're not. In any case, try to formulate your own plan for portion sizes.

CHAPTER ONE

Meats and Poultry

BLOOD TYPE A		Weekly, if your ancestry is . . .		
	PORTION	AFRICAN	CAUCASIAN	ASIAN
Lean red meats	4–6 oz. (men)	0–1 x	0–1 x	0–1 x
Poultry	2–5 oz. (women and children)	0–3 x	0–3 x	1–4 x

To receive the greatest benefits, Type As should eliminate all meats from your diet. Begin by substituting fish for meat several times a week. When you *do* eat meat, choose poultry over red meat. Prepare it by broiling or baking. Stay away from processed meat products like ham, frankfurters, and cold cuts. They contain nitrates, which promote stomach cancer in people with low levels of stomach acid—a Type A trait.

HIGHLY BENEFICIAL

None	

NEUTRAL

Chicken	Ostrich
Cornish hen	Squab
Grouse	Turkey
Guinea hen	

AVOID

Bacon/ham/pork	Mutton
Beef	Partridge
Buffalo	Pheasant
Duck	Quail
Goat	Rabbit
Goose	Squirrel
Heart/sweetbreads	Turtle
Horse	Veal
Lamb	Venison
Liver (Calf)	

CHAPTER TWO

Seafood

BLOOD TYPE A		Weekly, if your ancestry is . . .		
	PORTION	AFRICAN	CAUCASIAN	ASIAN
All seafood	4–6 oz.	1–3 x	1–3 x	1–3 x

Type As can eat seafood in modest quantity two or three times a week, but should avoid white fish like sole and flounder. They contain a lectin that can irritate the Type A digestive tract. If you are a Type A woman with a family history of breast cancer, I urge you to introduce snails into your diet. The edible snail *Helix pomatia* contains a powerful lectin that specifically agglutinates and is drawn to mutated Type A cells for two of the most common forms of breast cancer. This is a positive kind of agglutination; this lectin gets rid of sick cells.

HIGHLY BENEFICIAL

Carp	Red snapper
Cod	Salmon
Mackerel	Sardine
Monkfish	Snail
Perch (silver, yellow)	Trout (rainbow, sea)
Pickerel	Whitefish
Pollack	Whiting

NEUTRAL

Abalone	Mahimahi
Bass (sea)	Mullet
Bullhead	Muskellunge
Butterfish	Perch (ocean, white)
Chub	Orange roughy
Croaker	Parrot fish
Cusk	Pike
Drum	Pompano
Halfmoon fish	

NEUTRAL (CONTINUED)

Porgy	Sturgeon
Rosefish	Sucker
Sailfish	Sunfish
Salmon roe	Swordfish
Scrod	Tilapia
Sea bass	Trout (brook)
Shark	Tuna
Smelt	Weakfish
Snapper	Yellowtail

AVOID

Anchovy	Caviar
Barracuda	Clam
Bass (bluegill, striped)	Conch
Beluga	Crab
Bluefish	Crayfish
Catfish	Eel

AVOID (CONTINUED)

Flounder	Mollusks
Frog	Mussels
Gray sole	Octopus
Grouper	Opaleye fish
Haddock	Oyster
Hake	Scallop
Halibut	Scup
Harvest fish	Shad
Herring (fresh)	Shrimp
Herring (pickled)	Sole, all kinds
Lobster	Squid (calamari)
Lox	Tilefish

CHAPTER THREE

Eggs and Dairy

BLOOD TYPE A		Weekly, if your ancestry is . . .		
	PORTION	AFRICAN	CAUCASIAN	ASIAN
Eggs	1 egg	1–3 x	1–3 x	1–3 x
Cheese	2 oz.	0–2 x	1–3 x	0–2 x
Yogurt	4–6 oz.	0–1 x	1–3 x	0–3 x
Milk	4–6 oz.	0–1 x	1–3 x	0–3 x

Type As can tolerate small amounts of fermented dairy products, but should avoid anything made with whole milk, and also limit egg consumption to occasional organically grown eggs.

Your Type A choices should be yogurt, kefir, nonfat sour cream, and cultured dairy products. Raw goat's milk is a good substitute for whole milk.

If you are a Type A allergy sufferer or are experiencing respiratory problems, be aware that dairy products greatly increase the amount of mucus you secrete. Type As normally produce more mucus than the other blood types, but an overabundance of mucus inevitably leads to allergic responses, infections, and respiratory problems. This is another good reason to limit your intake of dairy foods.

HIGHLY BENEFICIAL

None	

NEUTRAL

Egg, chicken	Goat milk
Egg, duck	Kefir
Egg, goose	Mozzarella
Egg, quail	Paneer
Farmer cheese	Ricotta
Feta cheese	Sour cream (low/no fat)
Ghee (clarified butter)	Yogurt
Goat cheese	

AVOID

American cheese	Brie
Blue cheese	Butter

AVOID (CONTINUED)

Buttermilk	**Jarlsberg**
Camembert	**Milk (cow's)**
Casein	**Monterey jack**
Cheddar	**Muenster**
Colby	**Neufchâtel**
Cottage cheese	**Parmesan**
Cream cheese	**Provolone**
Edam	**Sherbet**
Emmenthal	**String cheese**
Gouda	**Swiss**
Gruyère	**Whey**
Half & Half	**Whole milk**
Ice cream	

CHAPTER FOUR

Oils and Fats

BLOOD TYPE A		Weekly, if your ancestry is . . .		
Oils	PORTION 1 tablespoon	AFRICAN 5–8 x	CAUCASIAN 5–8 x	ASIAN 5–8 x

Type As need very little fat to function well, but a tablespoon of olive oil on your salads or steamed vegetables every day will aid in digestion and elimination. As a monounsaturated fat, olive oil also has a positive effect on your heart and may actually reduce cholesterol.

HIGHLY BENEFICIAL

Black currant seed	Olive
Linseed (flaxseed)	Walnut

NEUTRAL

Almond	Safflower
Borage seed	Sesame
Canola	Soy
Cod-liver	Sunflower
Evening primrose	Wheat germ

AVOID

Castor	Cottonseed
Coconut	Peanut
Corn	

CHAPTER FIVE

Nuts and Seeds

BLOOD TYPE A		Weekly, if your ancestry is . . .		
	PORTION	AFRICAN	CAUCASIAN	ASIAN
Nuts and seeds	Small handful	4–7 x	4–7 x	4–7 x
Nut butters	1–2 tablespoons			

Since Type As eat very little animal protein, nuts and seeds supply an important protein component to your diet. Eat peanuts often because they contain a cancer-fighting lectin. Also eat the peanut skins. (The *skins,* not the shells.) If you have gallbladder problems, limit yourself to small amounts of nut butters instead of whole nuts.

HIGHLY BENEFICIAL

Flaxseed	Pumpkin seed
Peanut	Walnut
Peanut butter	

NEUTRAL

Almond	Macadamia nut
Almond butter	Pecan
Almond cheese	Pignola (pine nut)
Almond milk	Poppy seed
Beechnut	Safflower
Butternut	Sesame butter (tahini)
Chestnut	Sesame seed
Filbert (hazelnut)	Sunflower butter
Hickory nut	Sunflower seed
Lychee	

AVOID

Brazil nut	Pistachio
Cashew	

CHAPTER SIX

Beans and Legumes

BLOOD TYPE A		Weekly, if your ancestry is . . .		
Beans and legumes	PORTION 1 cup, dry	AFRICAN 5–7 x	CAUCASIAN 5–7 x	ASIAN 5–7 x

Type As thrive on the vegetable proteins found in beans and legumes. Many beans and legumes provide a nutritious source of protein. Be aware, however, that not *all* beans and legumes are good for you. Some, like kidney, lima, navy, and garbanzo, contain a lectin that can cause a decrease in insulin production, which is a factor in both obesity and diabetes.

Soy beans and their products—tofu, tempeh, soy milk, soy cheese—are highly recommended as Type A diet staples. Many supermarkets now carry these products, and they are available in health-food stores.

HIGHLY BENEFICIAL

Adzuki bean	Pinto bean
Black bean	Soy bean
Black-eyed pea	*Soy cheese
Fava bean	*Soy milk
Green bean	*Soy, tempeh
Lentil bean	*Soy, tofu
Soy, miso*	

soy products

NEUTRAL

Broad bean	Northern bean
Cannellini bean	Snap bean
Green pea	String bean
Jícama bean	White bean
Mung bean	

AVOID

Copper bean	Navy bean
Garbanzo bean (chickpea)	Red bean
Kidney bean	Tamarind bean
Lima bean	

CHAPTER SEVEN

Grains, Breads and Pasta

BLOOD TYPE A		Weekly, if your ancestry is . . .		
	PORTION	AFRICAN	CAUCASIAN	ASIAN
Grains, breads, and pasta	½ cup dry grains/ pasta, 1 muffin, 2 slices bread	7–10 x	7–9 x	7–10 x

Type As generally do well on cereals, as long as you select the more concentrated whole grains instead of instant and processed cereals. Stay away from instant products such as frozen meals, prepared noodles with sauces, or packaged rice and vegetable combinations. Instead, gain the full nutritional benefits from whole grain foods. If you have a pronounced mucous condition, asthma or frequent infections, limit your wheat consumption, as wheat causes mucous production. You'll have to experiment for yourself to determine how much wheat you can eat.

Breads and muffins are generally favorable foods, but observe the caveat about wheat, above. Soy and rice flour are good substitutes for you. Type As have a wonderful variety of choices in grains and pastas. These foods are excellent sources of vegetable protein. They can provide many of the nutrients lacking in your diet from the absence of animal proteins.

HIGHLY BENEFICIAL

Amaranth	Rice bran
Artichoke pasta (pure)	Rice cake
Buckwheat	Rice flour
Essene bread (manna bread)	Rye flour
Ezekiel 4:9 bread (100 percent sprouted)	Soba noodles (100 percent buckwheat)
Oat bread (100 percent whole oat)	
Oat flour	

NEUTRAL

Barley	Quinoa
Corn	Rice bran
Cornflakes	Rice bread
Cornmeal	Rice milk
Corn muffin	Rice, puffed
Couscous (cracked wheat)	Rice (white/brown/Basmati/wild)
Cream of rice	Rye bread (100 percent)
Fun crisp	Ry-krisp
Gluten flour	Rye vita
Grits	Sorghum
Ideal flat bread	Spelt flour/products
Kamut	Tapioca
Millet	Wheat (gluten flour products)
Oat bran/oatmeal	Wheat (refined, unbleached)
Popcorn	Wheat (semolina flour products)

NEUTRAL (CONTINUED)

Wheat (white flour products)	Wheat bread (sprouted commercial)
Wheat (whole wheat products)	

AVOID

Cream of Wheat	Matzo
English muffin	Wheat bran
Familia	Wheat germ
Farina	Shredded wheat
Grape-Nuts	

CHAPTER EIGHT

Vegetables

BLOOD TYPE A		Daily, if your ancestry is . . .		
	PORTION	AFRICAN	CAUCASIAN	ASIAN
Cooked	1 cup	Unlimited	Unlimited	Unlimited
Raw	1 cup	Unlimited	Unlimited	Unlimited

Vegetables are vital to the Type A diet, providing minerals, enzymes, and antioxidants. Eat your vegetables in as natural a state as possible (raw or steamed) to preserve their full benefits.

Most vegetables are available to Type As, but there are a few caveats: Peppers aggravate the delicate Type A stomach, as do the molds in fermented olives. Type As are also very sensitive to the lectins in domestic potatoes, sweet potatoes, yams, and cabbage. Avoid tomatoes, as their lectins have a negative effect on the Type A digestive tract. Broccoli is highly recommended for its antioxidant benefits. Antioxidants strengthen the immune system and prevent abnormal cell division. Other vegetables that are excellent for Type As are carrots, collard greens, kale, pumpkin, and spinach. Yellow onions are very good immune boosters, too. They contain a substance called quercitin, which is a powerful antioxidant.

Maitake mushrooms are revered in Japan as a powerful tonic for the immune system. Recent studies suggest that they may have anticancer properties.

HIGHLY BENEFICIAL

Alfalfa sprouts	Escarole
Aloe (plant, juice)	Fennel
Artichoke	Garlic
Beet greens	Ginger
Broccoli	Horseradish
Carrot/carrot juice	Kale
Celery/celery juice	Kohlrabi
Chicory	Leek
Collard greens	Lettuce, romaine
Dandelion	Mushroom, maitake

HIGHLY BENEFICIAL (CONTINUED)

Mushroom, silver dollar	Pumpkin
Okra	Rappini (broccoli rabe)
Onion (green, red, spanish, yellow)	Spinach/juice
Parsley	Swiss chard
Parsnip	Turnip

NEUTRAL

Arugula	Cabbage juice
Asparagus	Cauliflower
Asparagus pea	Celeriac
Avocado	Corn
Bamboo shoot	Cucumber/juice
Beet/beet greens/juice	Daikon radish
Bok choy	Endive
Brussels sprouts	Fiddlehead fern

NEUTRAL (CONTINUED)

Kelp	Radish sprouts
Lettuce (bibb/Boston/ butter/iceberg/mesclun/ radicchio)	Rutabaga
Mung bean sprouts	Scallion
Mushroom (abalone/ enoki/oyster/portabello/ straw)	Seaweed
Mustard greens	Senna
Olive, green	Shallot
Oyster plant	Squash (all types, except pumpkin)
Pea (green/pod/snow)	String bean
Pickles (in brine)	Taro
Pimiento	Water chestnut
Poi	Watercress
Radish	Zucchini

AVOID

Cabbage (not juice)	Potato, all types
Eggplant	Rhubarb
Juniper	Sauerkraut
Mushroom, shiitake	Sweet potato
Olive (black/Greek/ Spanish)	Tomato/juice
Peppers, all types	Yam
Pickles (in vinegar)	Yucca

CHAPTER NINE

Fruits

BLOOD TYPE A		Daily, if your ancestry is . . .		
Recommended fruits	PORTION 3–5 oz. or 1 fruit	AFRICAN 2–4 x	CAUCASIAN 3–4 x	ASIAN 3–4 x

Type As should eat fruits at least three times a day. Most fruits are allowable, although you should try to emphasize the more alkaline fruits, such as berries and melons, which can help to balance the acid-forming grains. Type As don't do well on tropical fruits like mangoes and papaya. Oranges should also be avoided, since they're a stomach irritant for Type As, and they also interfere with the absorption of important minerals. Grapefruit is closely related to oranges and is also an acidic fruit, but it has positive effects on the Type A stomach, exhibiting alkaline tendencies after digestion. Pineapple is an excellent digestive for Type As. Lemons are also excellent for Type As, aiding digestion and clearing mucus from the system. Since vitamin C is an important antioxidant, especially for stomach cancer prevention, eat other vitamin C–rich fruits, such as grapefruit or kiwi. The banana lectin interferes with Type A digestion. I recommend substituting other high-potassium fruits such as apricots, figs, and certain melons. Unless noted separately, all values of the whole fruit apply to the juice as well.

HIGHLY BENEFICIAL

Apricot	Grapefruit
Blackberry	Lemon
Blueberry	Lime
Boysenberry	Pineapple
Cherry, all types	Plum, all types
Cherry juice (black)	Prune
Fig, (fresh/dried)	

NEUTRAL

Apple/apple cider	Breadfruit
Asian pear	Canang melon

NEUTRAL (CONTINUED)

Cantaloupe	Nectarine
Casaba melon	Peach
Christmas melon	Pear
Cranberry/juice	Persian melon
Crenshaw melon	Persimmon
Currant, black and red	Pomegranate
Date	Prickly pear
Dewberry	Quince
Elderberry	Raisin
Gooseberry	Raspberry
Grape, all types	Sago palm
Guava	Spanish melon
Kiwi	Star fruit (carambola)
Kumquat	Strawberry
Loganberry	Watermelon
Musk melon	Youngberry

AVOID

Banana	**Orange**
Bitter melon	**Papaya**
Coconut/milk	**Plantain**
Honeydew melon	**Tangerine**
Mango	

CHAPTER TEN

Juices and Fluids

BLOOD TYPE A		Daily, if your ancestry is . . .		
	PORTION	AFRICAN	CAUCASIAN	ASIAN
Recommended juices	8 oz.	2–3 x	2–3 x	2–3 x
Lemon and water	8 oz.	morning	morning	morning
Water	8 oz.	4 +	4 +	4 +

Type As should start every day with a small glass of warm water into which you have squeezed the juice of one-half lemon. This will help you reduce the mucus that has accumulated overnight and stimulate normal elimination. Choose vegetables and fruits according to the recommendations in chapters 10 and 11 when making or buying juice. Alkaline fruit juices, such as black-cherry-juice concentrate diluted with water, should be consumed in preference to high-sugar juices, which are more acid forming.

CHAPTER ELEVEN

Spices

Type As should view spices as more than just flavor enhancers. The right combination of spices can be powerful immune system boosters. For example, soy-based spices like tamari, miso, and soy sauce are tremendously beneficial for Type As. If you're concerned about sodium intake, all of these products are available in low-sodium versions. Use plenty of garlic. It's a natural antibiotic and immune system booster, and it's good for your blood. Every blood type benefits from the use of garlic, but perhaps Type A benefits most of all, because your immune system is vulnerable to a number of diseases that garlic works against. Blackstrap molasses is a very good source of iron, a mineral that is lacking in the Type A diet. Kelp is an excellent source of iodine and many other minerals. Vinegar should be avoided because of its acidic properties.

Sugar and chocolate are allowed on the Type A Diet, but only in very small amounts. Use them as you would a condiment.

HIGHLY BENEFICIAL

Barley malt	Molasses
Blackstrap molasses	Parsley
Garlic	Soy sauce
Ginger	Tamari
Horseradish	Turmeric
Miso	

NEUTRAL

Agar	Basil
Allspice	Bay leaf
Almond extract	Bergamot
Anise	Brown rice syrup
Apple pectin	Caraway
Arrowroot	Cardamom

NEUTRAL (CONTINUED)

Carob	Guarana
Chervil	Honey
Chive	Juniper
Chocolate	Licorice root
Cilantro (coriander leaves)	Mace
Cinnamon	Maple syrup
Clove	Marjoram
Coriander	Mustard (dry)
Cornstarch	Nutmeg
Corn syrup	Oregano
Cream of tartar	Paprika
Cumin	Peppermint
Curry	Rice syrup
Dextrose	Rosemary
Dill	Saffron
Dulse	Sage
Fructose	Savory

NEUTRAL (CONTINUED)

Sea salt	Tapioca
Spearmint	Tarragon
Steria	Thyme
Sugar (white/brown)	Vanilla
Tamarind	Yeast (baker's or brewer's)

AVOID

Algae (blue-green)	MSG
Aspartame	Pepper (black/white)
Caper	Peppercorn/red flakes
Carrageenan	Sucanat
Chili powder	Vinegar, all types
Gelatin, plain	Wintergreen
Guargum (gum arabic)	

CHAPTER TWELVE

Condiments

You can eat small quantities of jam, and low-fat salad dressing, if it's made without vinegar. Vinegar-pickled foods have been linked to stomach cancer in people with low levels of stomach acid. Eliminate ketchup from your diet; Type As can't digest the tomato or the vinegar.

HIGHLY BENEFICIAL

Mustard (prepared; no wheat or vinegar)	

NEUTRAL

Jam (from acceptable fruits)	Jelly (from acceptable fruits)

NEUTRAL (CONTINUED)

Mustard (prepared, with vinegar)	Salad dressing (low fat, from acceptable ingredients)

AVOID

Ketchup	Pickle relish
Mayonnaise	Vinegar-pickled vegetables and fruits
Pickles	Worcestershire sauce

CHAPTER THIRTEEN

Herbs and Herbal Teas

Type As can benefit from herbs and herbal teas that rev up your immune system and promote cardiovascular health. For example, hawthorn is a cardiovascular tonic; aloe, alfalfa, burdock, and echinacea are immune system boosters; and green tea possesses important antioxidant characteristics. Herbs like ginger and slippery elm increase stomach acid secretion. A few drops of Gentian extract (*Gentiana lutea*) in warm water, taken 30 minutes before a meal, is a good digestive stimulant. Herbal relaxants, like chamomile and valerian root, help reduce stress.

HIGHLY BENEFICIAL

Alfalfa	Ashwagandha
Aloe	Burdock

HIGHLY BENEFICIAL (CONTINUED)

Chamomile	Holy basil
Dandelion	Larch arabinog alactan
Echinacea	Milk thistle
Fenugreek	Rose hip
Gentian	Slippery elm
Ginger	St. John's wort
Gingko biloba	Stone root
Ginseng (siberian)	Valerian
Hawthorn	

NEUTRAL

Chickweed	Horehound
Coltsfoot	Licorice root
Dong quai	Linden
Elderberry	Mulberry
Goldenseal (gargle or topical use only)	Mullein
Hops	Peppermint

NEUTRAL (CONTINUED)

Raspberry leaf	Strawberry leaf
Sage	Thyme
Sarsaparilla	Vervain
Senna	White birch
Shepherd's purse	White oak bark
Skullcap	Yarrow
Spearmint	

AVOID

Catnip	Red clover
Cayenne	Rhubarb
Chaparral	Sassafras
Comfrey	Yellow dock
Corn silk	

CHAPTER FOURTEEN

Miscellaneous Beverages

Red wine is good for Type As because of its positive cardiovascular effects. A glass of red wine every day is believed to lower the risk of heart disease for both men and women. Coffee may actually be *good* for Type As, in moderation. It increases your stomach acid and also has the same enzymes as those found in soy. Alternate coffee and green tea for the best combination of benefits. All other beverages on the list should be avoided, in favor of plain water.

HIGHLY BENEFICIAL

Coffee (regular/decaf)	Wine, red
Tea, green	

NEUTRAL

Wine, white	

AVOID

Beer	Soda, all types
Liquor, all distilled	Seltzer water
Tea, black (regular/decaf)	

CHAPTER FIFTEEN

Type A Supplement Advisory

Your Type A Plan also includes recommendations about vitamin, mineral, and herbal supplements that can enhance the effects of your diet. As with food, nutritional supplements don't always work the same way for everyone. Every vitamin, mineral, and herbal supplement plays a specific role in your body. The miracle remedy your Type B friend raves about may be inert or even harmful for your Type A system.

Your goal for supplement use should be to:

- Strengthen your immune system.

- Supply cancer-fighting antioxidants.

- Prevent infections.

- Improve your cardiovascular function.

BENEFICIAL

Vitamin B

Type As should be alert to vitamin B_{12} deficiency. Not only is the Type A Diet somewhat lacking in this nutrient, which is mostly found in animal proteins, but you tend to have a hard time absorbing the B_{12} you do eat because you lack intrinsic factor in your stomach. (Intrinsic factor is a substance produced by the lining of the stomach, which helps to absorb B_{12} into the blood.) In elderly Type As, vitamin B_{12} deficiency can cause senile dementia and other neurological impairments. Most other B vitamins are adequately contained in the Type A diet. If, however, you suffer from anemia, you may want a small supplement of folic acid. Type A heart patients should ask your doctors about low-dose niacin supplements, as niacin has cholesterol-lowering properties.

BEST B-RICH FOODS FOR TYPE A:
whole grains (niacin)
soy sauce (B_{12})
miso (B_{12})
tempeh (B_{12})

fish
_____

eggs
_____

Vitamin C

Type As, who have higher rates of stomach cancer because of low stomach acid, can benefit from taking additional supplements of vitamin C. For example, nitrate, a compound that results from the smoking and curing of meats, could be a particular problem for Type As because its cancer-causing potential is greater in people with lower levels of stomach acid. As an antioxidant, vitamin C is known to block this reaction (although you should still avoid smoked and cured foods). However, don't take this to mean that you should ingest massive amounts of vitamin C. I have found that Type As do not do as well on high doses (1000 mg and up) of vitamin C all at once, because it tends to upset your stomach. Taken over the course of a day, two to four capsules of a 250 mg supplement, preferably derived from rose hips, should cause no digestive problems.

BEST C-RICH FOODS FOR TYPE A:
berries
grapefruit
pineapple
cherries
lemon
broccoli

Vitamin E

There is some evidence that vitamin E serves as a protection against both cancer and heart disease—two Type A susceptibilities. You may want to take a daily supplement—no more than 400 IU (international units).

BEST E-RICH FOODS FOR TYPE A:
vegetable oil
whole grains
wheat germ
peanuts
leafy green vegetables

Calcium

A small amount of additional calcium (300–600 mg elemental calcium) from middle age onward is advisable for Type As. In my experience, the worst source of calcium for Type As is the simplest and most readily available: calcium carbonate (often found in antacids). This form requires the highest amount of stomach acid for absorption. In general, Type As tolerate calcium gluconate, do well on calcium citrate, and do best of all on calcium lactate.

BEST CALCIUM-RICH FOODS FOR TYPE A:

yogurt and other cultured dairy foods

soy milk

eggs

goat milk

canned salmon with bones

sardines with bones

broccoli

spinach

Iron

The Type A diet is naturally low in iron, which is found in the greatest abundance in red meats. Type A women, especially those with heavy menstrual periods, should be especially careful about keeping sufficient iron stores. If you need iron supplementation, do it under a doctor's supervision, so blood tests can monitor your progress. In general, use as low a dose as possible, and avoid extended periods of supplementation. Try to avoid crude iron preparations such as ferrous sulfate, which can irritate your stomach. Milder forms, such as iron citrate or blackstrap molasses, may be used instead. Floradix, a liquid iron and herbal supplement, can be found at most health-food stores and is readily assimilated by Type As.

BEST IRON-RICH FOODS FOR TYPE A:

whole grains

beans

figs

blackstrap molasses

Zinc [with caution]

I have found that a small amount of zinc supplementation (as little as 3 mg/day) often makes a big difference in protecting children against infections, especially
ear infections. Zinc supplementation is a double-edged
sword, however. While small, periodic doses enhance
immunity, long-term, higher doses depress it and can interfere with the absorption of other minerals. Be careful
with zinc! It's completely unregulated and is widely
available as a supplement, but you really shouldn't use
it without a physician's guidance.

BEST ZINC-RICH FOODS FOR TYPE A:

eggs

legumes

Selenium [with caution]

Selenium, which seems to act as a component of the
body's own antioxidant defenses, may be of value to
cancer-prone Type As. However, cases of selenium tox-
icity have been reported in people who have taken excessive supplements. Check with your physician before
taking selenium supplements on your own.

AVOID

Vitamin A (beta-carotene)

Recent studies suggest that beta-carotene in high doses may act as a pro-oxidant, speeding up damage to the tissues rather than stopping it. For this reason, Type As may wish to forgo beta-carotene supplements and consume high levels of carotenoids in their diet instead. Carotenoids are plentiful in the vegetable-based Type A diet—carrots in particular contain significant amounts. One caveat: as we age, our ability to assimilate the fat-soluble vitamins may diminish. Elderly Type As might benefit from small supplemental doses of vitamin A (10,000 IU daily) to help counteract the effects of aging upon the immune system.

BEST CAROTENE-RICH FOODS FOR TYPE A:
eggs
yellow squash
carrots
spinach
broccoli

HERBS/ PHYTOCHEMICALS

Hawthorn (*Crataegus oxyacantha*). Hawthorn is a great cardiovascular tonic. Type As should definitely add it to your diet regimen if you or members of your family have a history of heart disease. Hawthorn increases the elasticity of the arteries and strengthens the heart, while also lowering blood pressure and exerting a mild solventlike effect upon plaque in the arteries. Extracts and tinctures are readily available through naturopathic physicians, health-food stores, and pharmacies.

Immune-enhancing herbs. Type As tend to be open to immune-compromising infections, so gentle immune-enhancing herbs, such as purple coneflower (*Echinacea purpurea*), can help to ward off colds and the flu, and may help optimize your immune system's anticancer surveillance. Many people take echinacea in liquid or tablet form. It is widely available. The Chinese herb huangki (*Astragalus membranaceous*) is also taken as an immune tonic, but is not as easy to find. In both herbs, the active ingredients are sugars that stimulate proliferation of white blood cells, which act in defense of the immune system.

Calming herbs. Type As can use mild herbal relaxants, such as chamomile and valerian root for stress reduction. These herbs are available as teas and should be taken frequently. Valerian has a bit of a pungent odor, which actually becomes pleasing once you get used to it.

Quercetin. Quercetin is a bioflavonoid, found abundantly in vegetables, particularly yellow onions. Quercetin supplements are widely available in health-food stores, usually in capsules of 100–500 mg. Quercetin is a very potent antioxidant, many hundreds of times more powerful than vitamin E. It can make a substantial contribution to Type A cancer-prevention strategies.

Milk thistle (*Silybum marianum*). Like quercetin, milk thistle is an effective antioxidant with a special capacity to reach very high concentrations in the liver and bile ducts. Type As can suffer from disorders of the liver and gallbladder. If your family has any history of liver, pancreas, or gallbladder problems, consider adding a milk thistle supplement (easily found in most health-food stores) to your protocol. Cancer patients who are receiving chemotherapy should use a milk thistle supplement to help protect the liver from damage.

Bromelain (pineapple enzymes). Type As who suffer from bloating or other signs of poor absorption of protein should take a bromelain supplement. This enzyme has a moderate ability to break down dietary proteins, helping the Type A digestive tract assimilate proteins better.

Probiotics. If the Type A diet is new for you, you may find that adjusting to a vegetarian diet is uncomfortable and produces excessive gas or bloating. A probiotic supplement can counter this effect by supplying the "good" bacteria usually found in the healthy Type A digestive tract. Look for probiotic supplements high in bifidus factor. This strain of bacteria is best suited to the Type A system.

CHAPTER SIXTEEN

Medical Strategies

Modern science has presented the medical community with a bewildering array of medications, and all of them are being prescribed by well-meaning physicians worldwide. But have we been careful enough in our use of antibiotics and vaccines? How do you know which medications are best for you, for your family, for your children? Again, blood type holds the answer.

As a naturopathic physician, I try to avoid prescribing over-the-counter medications. In most cases, there are natural alternatives that work just as well or better—and they don't have some of the problematic side effects of many pharmaceutical preparations.

The following natural remedies are safe for Type A:

ARTHRITIS

alfalfa

boswella

calcium

epsom salt bath

rosemary tea soak

CONGESTION

licorice tea

mullein

nettle

vervain

CONSTIPATION

aloe vera juice

fiber

larch tree bark (ARA-6)

psyllium

slippery elm

COUGH

coltsfoot

horehound

linden

CRAMPS, GAS

chamomile tea

fennel tea

ginger

peppermint tea

probiotic supplement with bifidus factor

DIARRHEA

blueberries

elderberries

L. acidophilus (yogurt culture)

raspberry leaf

EARACHE

garlic-mullein-olive-oil eardrops

FEVER

feverfew

vervain

white willow bark

FLU

echinacea

elderberry (prevention)

garlic

goldenseal

arabinogalactan

rose hip tea

HEADACHE

chamomile

damiana

feverfew

valerian

white willow bark

INDIGESTION, HEARTBURN

bromelain

gentian

ginger

goldenseal

peppermint

MENOPAUSAL SYMPTOMS

Phytoestrogens derived from wild yams, alfalfa, and soy beans

(Avoid using conventional estrogen replacement because of cancer risk)

MENSTRUAL CRAMPS

Black cohosh

Jamaican dogwood

NAUSEA

ginger

licorice root tea

SINUSITIS

fenugreek

thyme

stone root

SORE THROAT

fenugreek tea gargle

goldenseal-root-and-sage-tea gargle

TOOTHACHE

crushed-garlic gum massage

oil-of-cloves gum massage

CHAPTER SEVENTEEN

Frequently Asked Questions

Do I have to make all of the changes at once for my Type A Diet to work?

No. On the contrary, I suggest you start slowly, gradually eliminating the foods that are not good for you and increasing those that are highly beneficial. Many diet programs urge you to plunge in headfirst and radically change your life immediately. I think it's more realistic and ultimately more effective if you engage in a learning process. Don't just take my word for it. You have to "learn" it in your body. Before you begin your Type A Diet, you may know very little about which foods are good or bad for you. You're used to making your choices according to your taste buds, family traditions, and fad diet books. Chances are you are eating some foods that are good for you, but the Type A Diet provides you with a powerful tool for making informed choices every time. Once you know what your optimal eating plan is, you have the freedom to veer from your diet on occasion. Rigidity is the enemy of joy; I certainly am not a proponent of it. The Type A Diet is designed to make you feel great, not miserable and deprived. Obviously, there are going to be times when common sense tells you to relax the rules a bit—such as when you're eating at a relative's house.

I'm Blood Type A and my husband is Blood Type O. How do we cook and eat together? I don't want to prepare two separate meals.

My wife, Martha, and I have exactly the same situation. Martha is Type O and I am Type A. We find that we can usually share about two-thirds of a meal. The main difference is in the protein source. For example, if we make a stir-fry, Martha might separately prepare some chicken while I'll add cooked tofu. Or if we're eating a pasta dish, Martha might add a little cooked ground beef to her portion. It has become relatively easy for us because we are quite familiar with the specifics of each other's Blood Type Diet. I suggest you refer to the comprehensive books *Eat Right 4 Your Type* and *Cook Right 4 Your Type* for information and suggestions for living happily in multiple-blood-type families. I know that people often worry that there might be too many differences between blood types to make it work—but think about it. There are over 200 foods listed for each diet—many of them compatible across the board. Considering that the average person eats only about 25 foods, the Blood Type Diets actually offer more, not fewer, options.

Why do you list different portion recommendations according to ancestry?

The portions listings according to ancestry are merely refinements to the diet that you may find helpful. In the same way that men, women, and children have different portion standards, so, too, do people according to their body size and weight, geography, and cultural food preferences. These suggestions will help you get started until you are comfortable enough with the diet to naturally eat the appropriate portions. The portion recommendations also take into account specific problems that people of different ancestries tend to have with food. African Americans, for example, are often lactose intolerant, and most Asians are unaccustomed to eating dairy foods, so the Type Bs among them, for example, may have to introduce these foods slowly to avoid negative reactions.

Must I eat all of the foods marked "highly benefi-cial"?

It would be impossible to eat everything on your diet! Think of your Blood Type Diet as a painter's palette from which you may choose colors in different shades and combinations. However, do try to reach the weekly frequency of the various food groups, if possible. Frequency is probably more important than the individual portions. If you have a small build, reduce the size of your portions, but maintain a regular frequency. This will ensure that the most valuable nutrients will continue to be delivered into the bloodstream at a constant rate.

What should I do if an "avoid" food is the fourth or fifth ingredient in a recipe?

That depends on the severity of your condition, or the degree of your compliance. If you have food allergies, or colitis, you may want to practice complete avoidance. Many high-compliance patients avoid these foods altogether, although I think this might be too extreme. Unless you suffer from a specific allergic condition, it won't hurt most people to occasionally eat a food that is not on their diet.

Will I lose weight on the Blood Type Diet?

There are several ways to answer that question. First, most people who are overweight are eating an imbalanced diet—foods that upset metabolism, hamper proper digestion, and cause water retention. These are all factors that lead to overweight. The Blood Type Diet is the ultimate *balanced* diet, specifically tailored for you. If you follow your Blood Type Diet, your metabolism will adjust to its normal level and you'll burn calories more efficiently; your digestive system will process nutrients properly and reduce water retention. In time, perhaps a very short time, your weight will adjust accordingly. In my practice, I've found that most of my patients who have weight problems also have a history of chronic dieting. One would think that constant dieting would lead to weight loss, but that's not true if the structure of the diet and the foods it includes go against everything that makes sense for your specific body type. In our culture, we tend to promote "one size fits all" weight-loss programs, and then we wonder why they don't work. The answer is obvious! Different blood types respond to food in different ways. For example, Type As process bread and pasta more effectively than Type Os, but the animal protein they eat tends to be stored as fat. If you want to lose weight, your Blood Type Diet will tell you how. In conjunction with the recommended exercise program, you should see results very quickly.

Do calories matter on the Blood Type Diet?

There is an adjustment period on this diet, and over time you'll be able to adjust food amounts according to your needs. It's important to be aware of portion sizes. No matter *what* you eat, if you eat *too much* of it you'll gain weight. This probably seems so obvious that it doesn't even bear mentioning. But overeating has become one of America's most difficult and dangerous health problems. Millions of Americans are bloated and dyspeptic because of the amounts of food they eat. When you eat excessively, the walls of your stomach stretch like an inflated balloon. Although stomach muscles are elastic and were created to contract and expand, when they are grossly enlarged the cells of the abdominal walls undergo a tremendous strain. If you are eating until you feel full, and you normally feel sluggish after a meal, try to reduce your portion sizes. Learn to listen to what your body is telling you.

Tofu seems like a very unappealing food. Must I eat it if I'm Type A?

Many Type As are initially put off by the idea of tofu. Well, tofu is not a glamour food. I admit it. (When I was an impoverished Type A college student, I ate tofu with vegetables and brown rice almost every day for years. I actually liked it—sorry.) I think the real problem with tofu is the way it is usually displayed in the markets. Tofu—in soft or hard cakes—sits with its other tofu friends in a large plastic tub, immersed in cold water. If they can overcome their initial aversion and actually purchase one or two tofu "cakes," many people take it home, pop it on a plate, and break off a hunk to give it a try. This is a bad way to experience tofu! (Not unlike tossing a whole raw egg into your mouth and chewing . . . not very appealing.) If you are going to use tofu, it is best cooked and combined with vegetables and strong flavors that you enjoy, such as garlic, ginger, and soy sauce. Tofu is a nutritionally complete meal that is extremely inexpensive. Type As take note: The path to your good health is paved with bean curd!

I've never heard of many of the grains you mention. Where do I find out more?

If you're looking for alternative grains, health-food stores are a bonanza. In recent years, many ancient grains, largely forgotten, have been rediscovered and are now being produced. Examples of these are amaranth, a grain from Mexico, and spelt, a variation of wheat that seems to be free of the problems found with whole wheat. Try them! They're not bad. Spelt flour makes a hearty, chewy bread that is quite flavorful, while several interesting breakfast cereals are now being made with amaranth. Another alternative is to use sprouted wheat breads, sometimes referred to as "Ezekiel" or "Essene" bread, as the gluten lectins found principally in the seed coat are destroyed by the sprouting process. These breads spoil rapidly and are usually found in the refrigerator cases of health-food stores. They are a "live" food, with many beneficial enzymes still intact. (Beware of commercially produced "sprouted wheat" breads, as they usually have a minority of sprouted wheat and a majority of whole wheat in their formulas.) Sprouted wheat breads are somewhat sweet tasting, as the sprouting process also releases sugars, and are moist and chewy. They make wonderful toast.

Should I be concerned about the yeast in bread?

Many people worry that the yeast content of breads will cause problems, especially if they suffer from irritable bowel syndrome. Frankly, I have not seen this as a problem. I think what many people suspect to be a reaction to the yeast in bread is actually a reaction between the gluten lectins and the blood type chemicals in their digestive tract. I believe this to be the case because these patients usually tolerate high-yeast breads that are made of grains that are acceptable for their blood type. Other more common grains that work well as alternatives to corn and wheat are brown rice, rye, millet, oats, buckwheat, and wild rice.

I've begun to incorporate many of your recommendations and have seen marked differences in my health. My question is, how can peanuts be healthy if they contain aflatoxin?

Recently, a well-known figure in alternative medicine made several statements that cast doubt upon the safety of commercially available peanuts. As an answer to the question "Does peanut butter cause cancer?" the authority answered that "it's relatively common for aflatoxin to cause a type of poisoning called aflatoxicosis." This assertion is questionable at best. There are no reported incidences of aflatoxicosis in the United States contained in MEDLINE, the medical database, and only a few isolated instances in Third World countries (Uganda, 1971; India, 1975; and Malaysia, 1991), where methods of storage and identification are suspect. Indeed, even in the case of these reported "outbreaks" none was associated with peanut consumption! In Uganda and India the cause was contaminated corn, and in Malaysia a type of noodle. This does not sound "relatively common" to me, nor does it directly implicate peanuts as a dangerous source of aflatoxin any more than corn or walnuts.

In the United States, the FDA regulates aflatoxin, and it can be avoided or minimized with proper agricultural and manufacturing practices. Aflatoxins are highly controlled in food products for consumption and the concern for safety has been reduced drastically. The FDA's efforts to ensure the safety and quality of foods and feeds are complemented by control programs carried out by USDA, state departments of agriculture, and various industrial trade associations.

My children, ages five and seven, are reluctant to try new things. They're both Type A, and I have difficulty getting them to switch from milk to soy and from wheat to nonwheat foods. Any suggestions?

The best approach with children is to incorporate changes in a slow, gradual process. The most important area to focus on in the beginning is incorporating more of the beneficial Type A foods. Be patient about gradually reducing milk and wheat. Remember that food preferences are learned. Studies have shown that children, left to their own devices, select over the course of several weeks as good or better foods as those their parents would have picked for them. The watchwords therefore are . . . exposure to new foods and patience.

Type A at a Glance

TYPE A
The Cultivator
settled · copperative · orderly

STRENGTHS	WEAKNESSES	MEDICAL RISKS
Adapts well to dietary and environmental variety	Unable to digest and metabolize meat protein easily	Heart disease
		Type I and Type II diabetes
System preserves and metabolizes nutrients efficiently	Vulnerable immune system, open to microbial invasion	Cancer
		Liver and gallbladder disorders

DIET PROFILE	WEIGHT LOSS KEY	SUPPLEMENTS	EXERCISE REGIMEN
VEGETARIAN	AVOID	Vitamin B_{12}	Calming,
	Meat	Folic acid	centering
Vegetables	Dairy	Vitamin C	exercises,
Tofu	Kidney bean	Vitamin E	such as
Seafood	Lima bean	Hawthorn	yoga and
Grains	Wheat	Echinacea	Tai Chi
Beans		Quercetin	
Legumes	USE	Milk thistle	
Fruit	Olive oil		
	Soy foods		
	Seafood		
	Vegetables		
	Pineapple		

Blood Type Learning Center

Now that you're familiar with the basic principles of the Blood Type Diet, I encourage you to expand your level of learning and application. The "right for your type" series offers the most comprehensive, scientifically grounded, and clinically tested information available on the four blood types. In order to truly make the most of your individualized diet and lifestyle recommendations, it's important for you to have a working knowledge of all four blood types. Your differences do not exist in a vacuum, but are part of nature's complex system of opposition and synergism. Your understanding of the evolutionary factors that distinguish the blood types will enhance your ability to live more fully as a Type A. In addition, these books offer extensive additional information and recommendations about your blood type. The series includes:

Live Right 4 Your Type
The Individualized Prescription for
Maximizing Health, Metabolism, and
Vitality in Every Stage of Your Life
by Dr. Peter J. D'Adamo, with Catherine Whitney
(G. P. Putnam's Sons, 2001)
Also available on audiocassette

In *Live Right 4 Your Type*, Dr. D'Adamo shows how living according to blood type can help people achieve total physical and emotional health at every stage of life. Aided by cutting-edge genetic research and the documentation of hundreds of research studies, Dr. D'Adamo presents readers with a life-enhancing program, which includes:

- The latest discoveries about the genetics of blood type and how they affect the body's systems.

- A study of the role of subtypes, in particular secretor status.

- Groundbreaking data on the connection between blood type and stress, personality, and mental health.

- A thorough investigation of the variations in digestion, metabolism, and immunity, depending on blood type.

- Individualized blood type prescriptions that show how to make lifestyle adaptations, reduce stress, gain emotional balance, slow down aging, and avoid disease.

- Targeted advice for children, seniors, and women.

- Extensive research notes, patient outcomes, and resources.

Eat Right 4 Your Type
The Individualized Diet Solution to
Staying Healthy, Living Longer &
Achieving Your Ideal Weight
by Dr. Peter J. D'Adamo, with Catherine Whitney
(G. P. Putnam's Sons, 1996)
Also available on audiocassette

Eat Right 4 Your Type is Dr. D'Adamo's groundbreaking book, which first introduced the concept of the connection between blood type, diet, and health to a mass audience. With over two million copies in print and translated into fifty languages, *Eat Right 4 Your Type* remains the seminal work in the field. It includes:

- A detailed exploration of the anthropological and biological origins of the blood types.

- Comprehensive diet, exercise, and meal plans for each blood type.

- Special recommendations for medical problems, weight loss, aging, infertility, and other issues.

- Case histories from Dr. D'Adamo's clinic, showing the remarkable results of the Blood Type Diet.

- An extensive bibliography, research and support section.

Cook Right 4 Your Type
The Practical Kitchen Companion to
Eat Right 4 Your Type
by Dr. Peter J. D'Adamo, with Catherine Whitney
(G. P. Putnam's Sons, 1998)

Cook Right 4 Your Type is the essential guide for living with and enjoying your Blood Type Diet. With the assistance of a team of professional chefs, Dr. D'Adamo presents a book chock-full of vital information and delicious recipes for each blood type. The book features:

- Food lists and shopping guides to help you set up your kitchen.

- Family-friendly recipe charts that show how to cook for more than one blood type.

- Hundreds of tips and practical guidelines for eating right for your type.

- 30-day meal plans to help integrate the diet into daily life.

- More than 200 original recipes to please every blood type palate.

Resources and Support

DR. PETER J. D'ADAMO: PATIENT SERVICES

Dr. Peter D'Adamo and his staff continue to accept new patients on a limited basis. To find out more about scheduling an appointment, please contact:

The D'Adamo Clinic
2009 Summer Street
Stamford, CT 06905
203-348-4800

Note: Please do not submit questions regarding Dr. D'Adamo's work or seeking personal advice on health matters.

ON THE WEB: WWW.DADAMO.COM

The World Wide Web has proven to be a valuable venue for exploring and applying the tenets of the Blood Type Diet and lifestyle. Since January 1997 hundreds of thousands have visited the site to participate in the ABO chat groups, to peruse the scientific archives, to share experiences and recipes, and to learn more about the science of blood type. The Web site has an interactive message board and archives of past posts to the board.

One of the most important features on the Web page is the Blood Type Outcome Registry, which has facilitated the collection of data on the measurable effects of the Blood Type Diet on a wide range of medical conditions. Visitors are encouraged to share their results.

SELF-TESTING SERVICES

North American Pharmacal, Inc., is the official distributor of Home Blood Type Testing Kits. Each kit costs $7.95 and is a single-use disposable educational device capable of determining one individual's ABO and rhesus blood type. Results are obtained within four to five minutes. If you have several friends or family members who need to learn their blood type, you will need to order a separate home blood-typing kit for each individual.

All U.S. orders are shipped via UPS ground (shipping

and handling cost is $5.25 per order irrespective of the number of kits ordered). Expedited shipping methods (UPS second day or next day) are available but cost more. Please contact the customer-service department to inquire about rates for expedited shipping to your area.

If you are ordering a kit to be shipped outside of the U.S., shipping rates can vary dramatically and can be quite expensive. Please contact our customer-service department prior to placing your order for an estimate of shipping charges for non-U.S. orders.

To order a single Home Blood Typing Kit please enclose $7.95 + $5.25 for shipping and handling and send to:

North American Pharmacal, Inc.
5 Brook Street
Norwalk, CT 06851
Tel: 203-866-7664
Fax: 203-838-4066
Toll free: 877-ABO TYPE (877-226-8973)
www.4yourtype.com

North American Pharmacal, Inc., offers a range of other self-tests to monitor aspects of health such as stress hormone levels, female hormone levels, mineral balance, and antioxidant status. There is also a test to determine secretor status. For prices and ordering information please contact North American Pharmacal.

BLOOD TYPE PRODUCTS AND SUPPLEMENTS

North American Pharmacal, Inc., is the official distributor of Blood Type Specialty Products. The product line includes supplements, books, tapes, teas, meal replacement bars, cosmetics, and support material that makes eating and living right for your type easier. Included in this product line are: New Chapter® D'Adamo 4 Your Type Products™. These whole-food vitamins, herbs, and other food supplements have been specifically crafted to address the unique requirements of each blood type.

Also included are Sip Right 4 Your Type™ teas, Deflect™ lectin-blocking formulas, and a range of additional blood-type-specific and blood-type-friendly health products that have been formulated in partnership with The Republic of Tea and New Chapter.

Product information and price lists are available from:

North American Pharmacal, Inc.
5 Brook Street
Norwalk, CT 06851
Tel: 203-866-7664
Fax: 203-838-4066
Toll free: 877-ABO-TYPE (877-226-8973)
www.4yourtype.com